Learning With Colors
MEAT
to Grow On

by

Doris Cambruzzi and Claire Thornton

illustrations by Lorraine Arthur

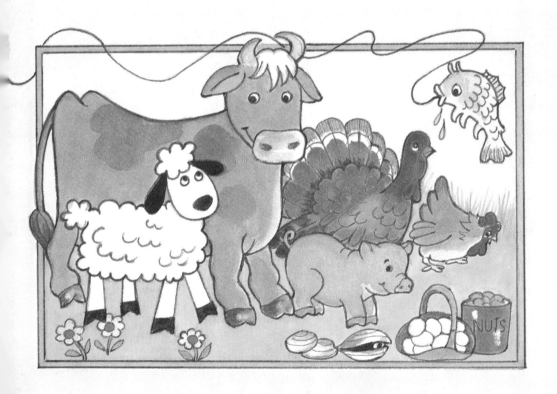

STANDARD PUBLISHING
Cincinnati, Ohio   3608

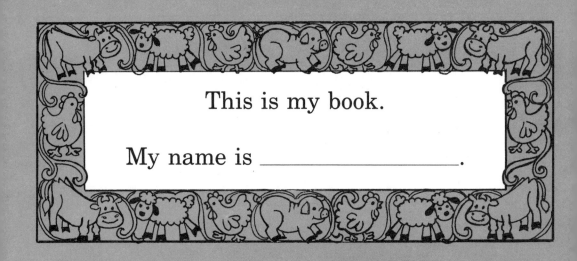

This is my book.

My name is _____.

Library of Congress Catalog Card Number 86-060738
ISBN 0-87403-128-1

Dear Parent:

God, our loving Father, has entrusted our children to us, to guide and direct in both spiritual and bodily growth here on earth. This book is designed to help your children become familiar with good nutrition so that they will eat the correct foods for a healthy body.

Nutrition pertains to what we eat and how our bodies use it. Essential nutrients must be obtained from the foods we eat. Protein, carbohydrates, fat, vitamins, minerals, and water are the six classes of essential nutrients we obtain from our diets.

Whether we eat at home or we eat out, we are faced with important food choices. Children's needs change with age. One set of rules simply cannot apply to everyone. There is a practical guide to good nutrition, which translates the technical knowledge of nutrition into a plan for everyday eating. This guide, "The Four Good Groups," provides the kind and quantity of food necessary for a balanced diet. The Four Food Groups are Fruit-Vegetable Group, Meat Group, Milk Group, and Bread-Cereal Group.

A key to good health is to eat a variety of foods from each of the four food groups every day and get proper rest and exercise. It is very important to start your young children with good health habits.

Why do some people accept some foods and reject others? A primary factor in food acceptance seems to be the training of the young child in familiarity with a wide variety of foods. This training should be started at an early age, supported both in the home and by effective educational experiences.

Coauthor Doris Cambruzzi conducted a study on this subject and found that education, in addition to the provision of food, was an important factor in the vegetable consumption practices of children. The pattern of eating established during early childhood is believed to affect food choice and, to some extent, nutritional status throughout life.

This book is a learning aid to help your child become familiar with foods from the Meat Group and to understand the correct portion that is needed by the body, which is the key to weight control throughout life. The illustrations of meat, fish, and poultry contained in this book will help children identify them, and the recipes are easy and fun.

—*Doris Cambruzzi*
—*Claire Thornton*

EAT A VARIETY OF FOODS FROM

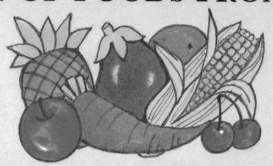

FRUIT-VEGETABLE
GROUP

Eat 4 or more servings each day from the Fruit-Vegetable Group. Foods in this group supply most of our daily needs for vitamin C and vitamin A. Fiber is present in all fruits and vegetables, especially in the skins.

One serving from the
Fruit-Vegetable Group

= ½ cup of a fruit or
vegetable, or a portion
as ordinarily served
such as 1 medium banana

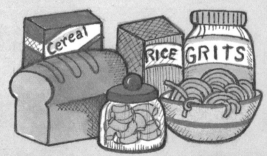

BREAD-CEREAL
GROUP

Eat 4 or more servings each day from the Bread-Cereal Group. Foods in this group supply many of the vitamins in the B complex, iron, carbohydrates, and limited amounts of protein. Fiber is present in whole grains.

One serving from the
Bread-Cereal Group

= 1 slice of bread
= 1 ounce of ready-to-eat cereal
= ½ to ¾ cup of cooked
cereal, macaroni, rice,
grits, or spaghetti

THE FOUR FOOD GROUPS!

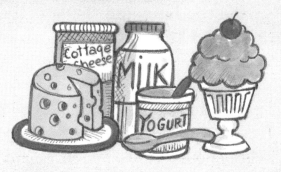

MILK GROUP

Drink or eat 2 to 3 servings daily of foods from the Milk Group if you are under age 9. This group is a primary source of calcium. It also gives us phosphorous, riboflavin (vitamin B_2), and complete protein.

One serving from the Milk Group

= 1 cup (8 ounces) of milk
= 1½ ounces of cheese
= 1¾ cups of ice cream
= 2 cups of cottage cheese
= 1 cup of yogurt

Lowfat and skim milk products have the same amount of calcium as whole milk, but not as many calories.

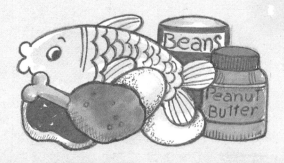

MEAT GROUP

Turn the page and have fun with the Meat Group.

God made us, and God made the food we eat. God made the land and the sea, the sun and the moon, the rain and the air around us, and all the animals and plants for us to enjoy.

Meat, fish, and poultry are some of the foods that God gave us to eat. They taste good and are good for us.

God wants us to have healthy bodies and to take good care of our bodies. When we eat the right foods, we grow and feel good; and when we feel good, we can serve Him better.

This book tells you about meat, fish, and poultry and gives you some recipes so that you can enjoy eating them in different ways. You will also learn to identify the many colors that make our world so beautiful.

Have fun eating foods from the Meat Group; they will help you stay healthy!

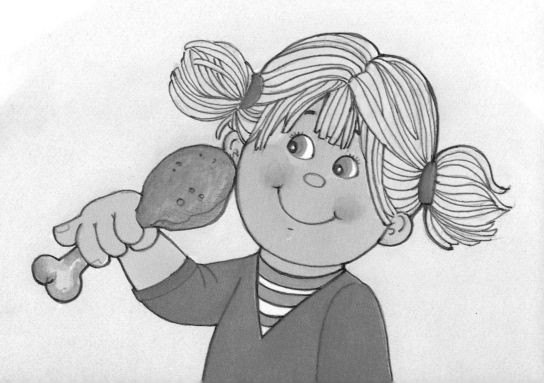

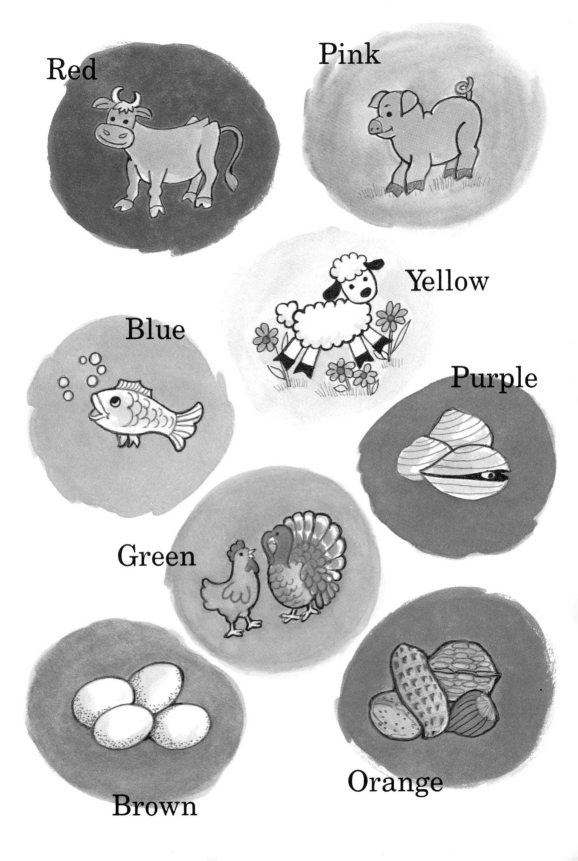

Red

Pink

Yellow

Blue

Purple

Green

Brown

Orange

MEAT GROUP

The Meat Group includes

Meat: Poultry
  beef   Eggs
  veal   Legumes:
  pork   dry beans and seeds
  lamb   peas
  wild game   lentils
Fish and shellfish   peanuts
                  nuts

Foods in the Meat Group are our main source of protein. They also contain B vitamins and iron. Only foods from animals contain vitamin B_{12}.

Iron keeps us from getting too tired. Iron is used best by the body when meats are eaten with foods containing vitamin C (such as lettuce and tomatoes on meat sandwiches or orange juice with eggs for breakfast).

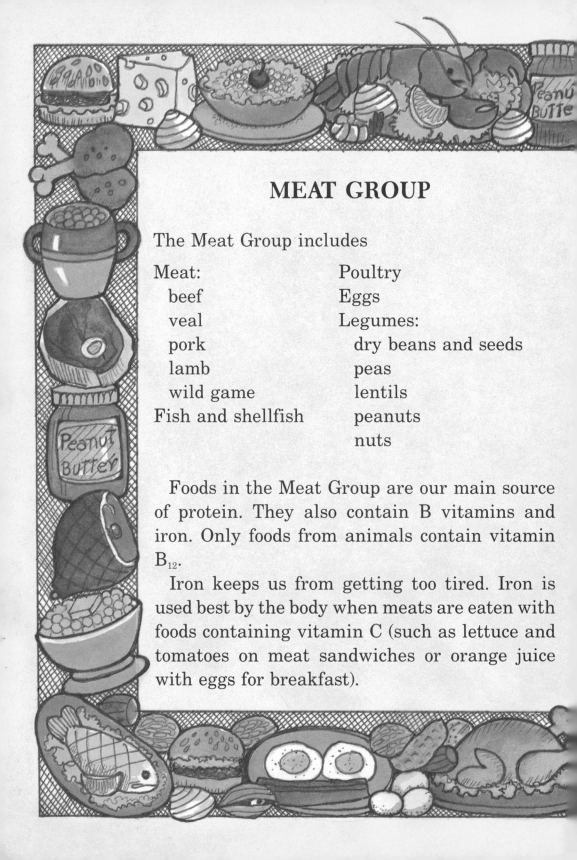

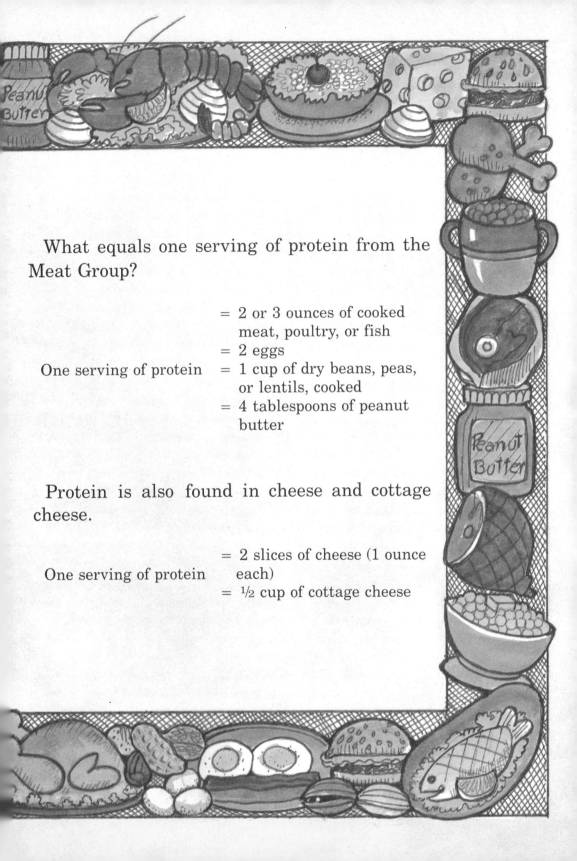

What equals one serving of protein from the Meat Group?

One serving of protein
= 2 or 3 ounces of cooked meat, poultry, or fish
= 2 eggs
= 1 cup of dry beans, peas, or lentils, cooked
= 4 tablespoons of peanut butter

Protein is also found in cheese and cottage cheese.

One serving of protein
= 2 slices of cheese (1 ounce each)
= ½ cup of cottage cheese

BEEF

RED

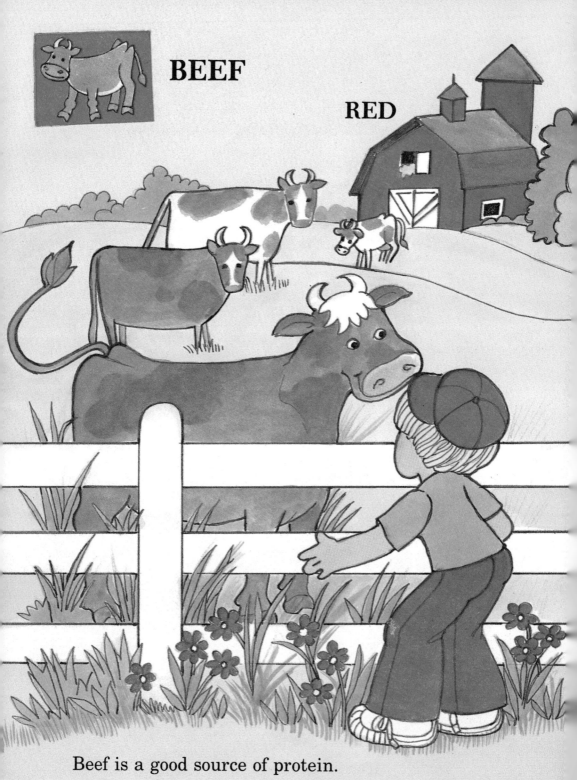

Beef is a good source of protein.

Beef comes from cows.

Sloppy Joes

1 pound ground beef
I tablespoon chopped onion
1 tablespoon vegetable oil
1 8-ounce can tomato sauce
4 tablespoons catsup
4 hamburger buns, cut in half

Cook onion in heated oil in skillet over medium heat.
When onion is clear, add ground beef.
Cook, stirring often until ground beef is no longer pink.
Add catsup and tomato sauce.
Stir mixture and cook until bubbling hot.
Spoon over bottom halves of buns,* and cover with top halves.
Makes 4 servings.

*If desired, toast buns under the broiler in the oven before filling with Sloppy Joe mixture.

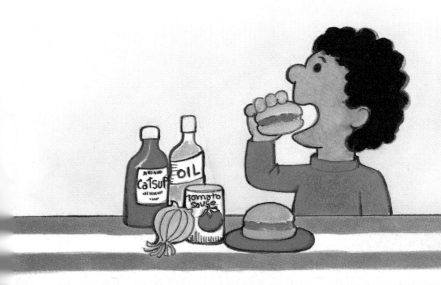

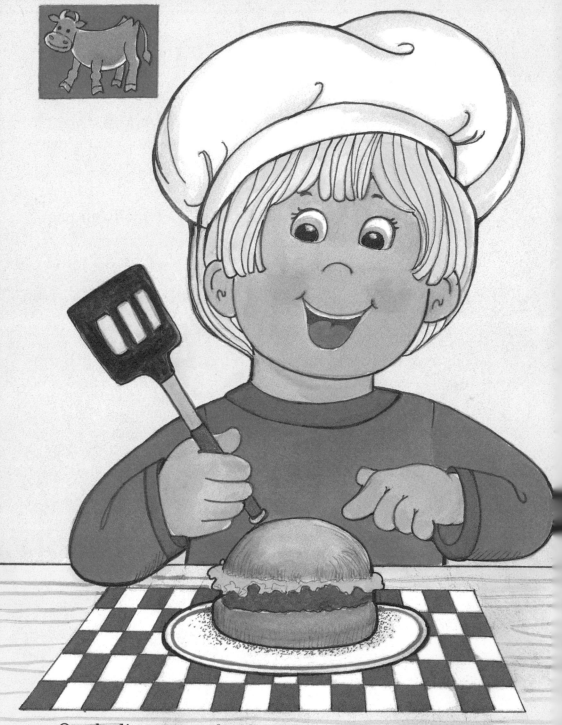

Our bodies are made of many tiny parts called cells.
Cells are made of protein.
Eating hamburgers gives us protein.

Hamburgers

1 pound ground beef
1 teaspoon salt
¼ teaspoon pepper
1 teaspoon minced onion
4 hamburger buns, split in half

Mix all the ingredients together in a medium-sized bowl.

Divide hamburger mixture into 4 parts.

Shape into round patties.

Cook hamburgers in a skillet on medium heat or in the oven under the broiler.

Buns can be toasted by placing them cut side up on a cookie sheet and putting them under the broiler until golden brown.

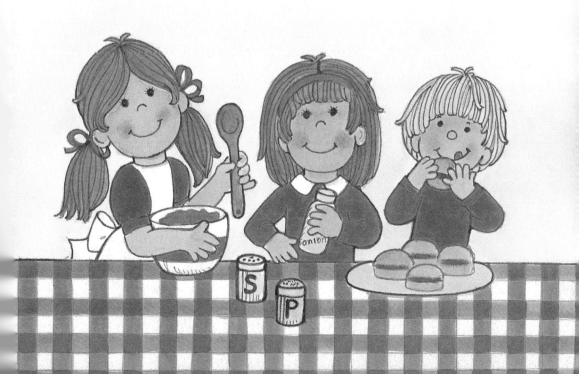

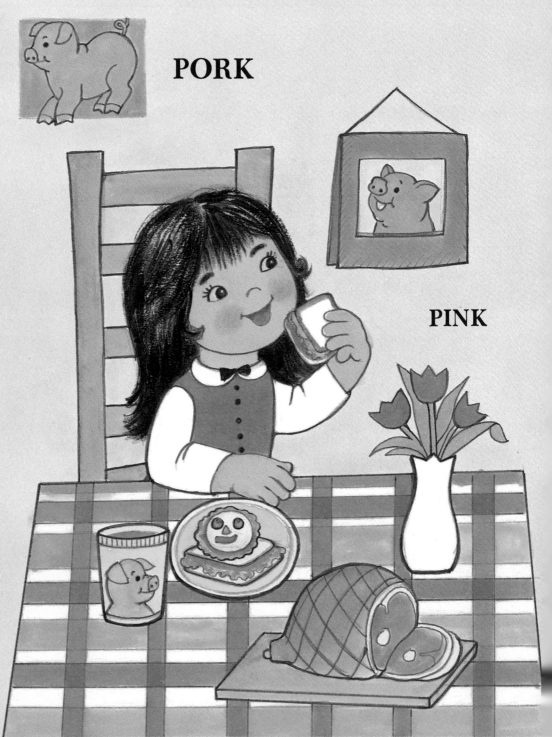

PORK

PINK

Pork is a good source of protein.
Pork and ham come from pigs.

Make-a-Face Ham Sandwiches

6 slices of ham
6 slices of white bread
6 slices of rye bread
Lettuce, mayonnaise
Raisins, nuts, carrot sticks, sliced stuffed olives, hard-
    boiled egg, and cheese slices for garnish

With a round cookie cutter or top of a glass, cut out circles of bread and make sandwiches, using ham, lettuce, and mayonnaise.

To make funny faces, cut each sandwich in half and put the eyes and nose on one half and the mouth on the other half, using garnishes.

For more fun, mix and match the halves.

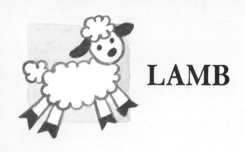

LAMB

YELLOW

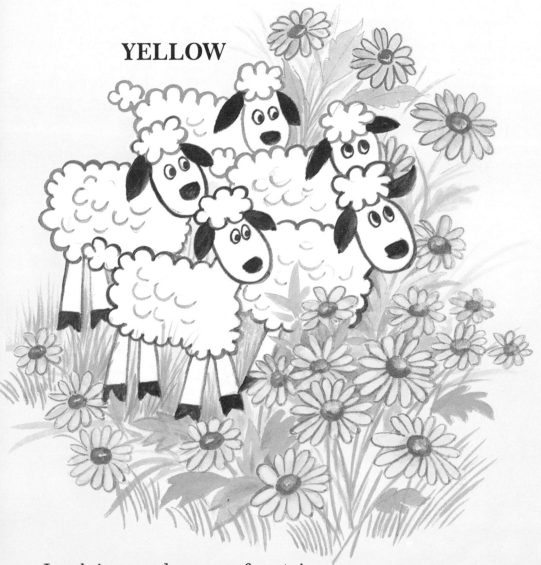

Lamb is a good source of protein.

Lamb comes from sheep.

Lamb Patties

1 pound ground lamb
4 slices onion
4 tablespoons catsup
Salt and pepper to taste

Divide the lamb into four equal parts and form into round patties.

Shake salt and pepper over the tops.

Press an onion slice onto the top of each patty, then spoon on a tablespoon of catsup.

Place on a broiler pan or shallow baking dish and bake in a 325 degree preheated oven for 20 minutes or until meat is no longer pink in the center.

Serves 4.

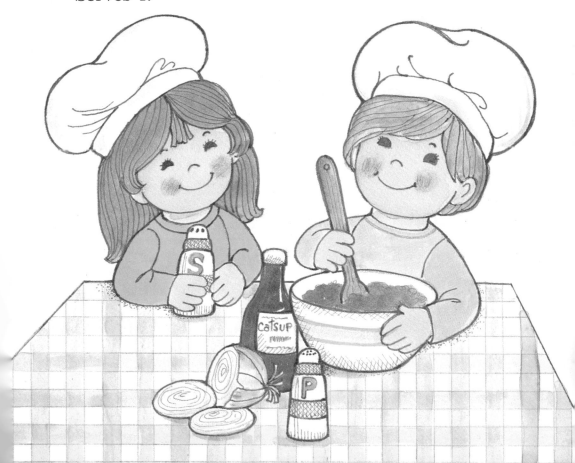

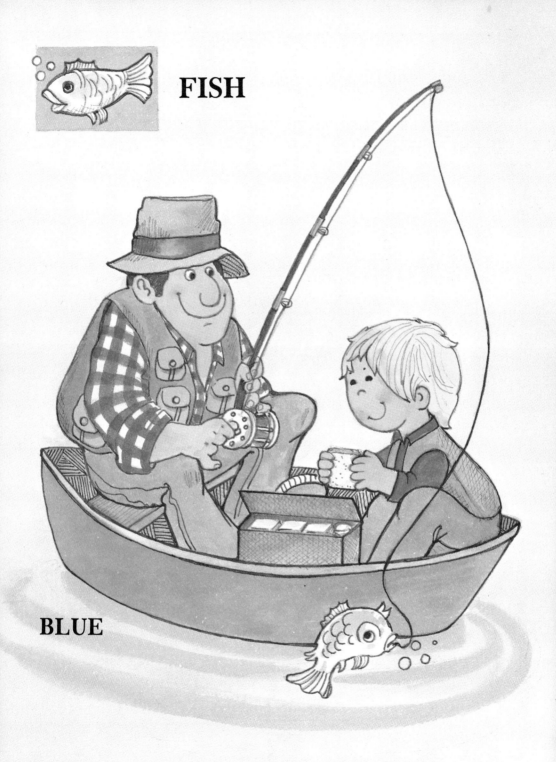

FISH

BLUE

Fish is a good source of protein.

Fish live in lakes, rivers, and oceans.

Tuna Salad in Pita Pockets

1 can tuna fish (6½ ounces)
4 tablespoons mayonnaise
4 tablespoons plain yogurt
2 tablespoons pickle relish
2 tablespoons chopped celery
2 tablespoons chopped onion
Dash pepper
Lettuce
4 slices of tomato

2 pita-bread rounds, cut in half crosswise

Mix tuna, mayonnaise, yogurt, pickle relish, chopped celery, and onion.

Add a dash of pepper to taste, and spoon into pita-bread pockets that have been lined with lettuce and a tomato slice.

Makes 4 tuna salad pita sandwiches.

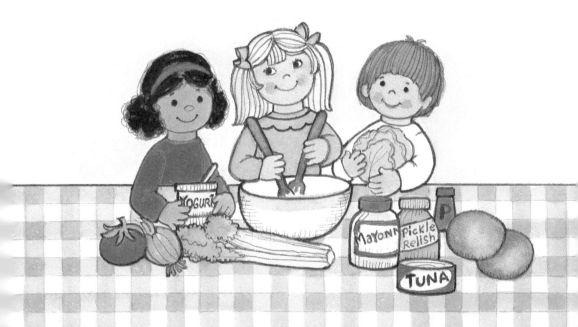

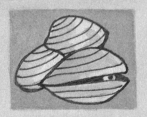

SHELLFISH

PURPLE

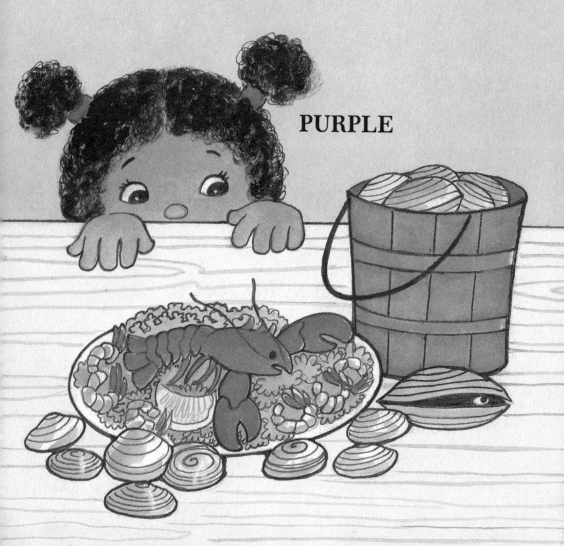

Shellfish such as shrimp, lobsters, and oysters live in salt water.

Shrimp Dip

1 package (3 ounces) cream cheese
1 cup commercial sour cream
1 can (5 ounces) shrimp
2 tablespoons onion, finely chopped
1 teaspoon Worchestershire sauce
¼ teaspoon salt

Blend cream cheese and sour cream with a fork or in a blender until fluffy.

Add remaining ingredients and blend gently but firmly.

Chill 2 hours to blend flavors.

Makes about 2 cups.

Serve as a dip with vegetable slices or whole-wheat crackers.

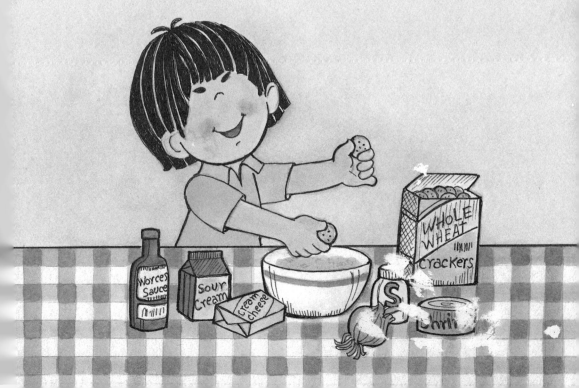

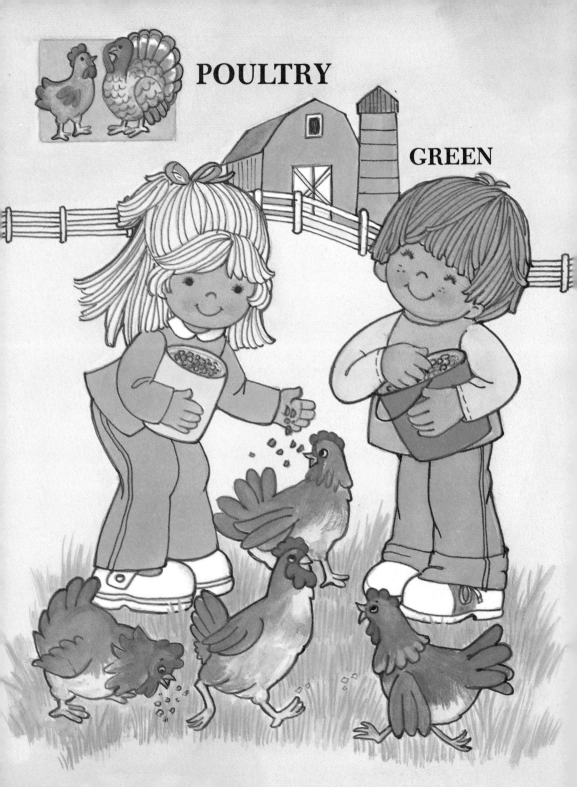

POULTRY

GREEN

Chicken and turkey are good sources of protein.

Oven-Fried Chicken

½ cup flour
1 teaspoon salt
¼ teaspoon pepper
2 teaspoons paprika
½ cup vegetable shortening

2- to 3-pound frying chicken, cut up

Mix flour, salt, pepper, and paprika in paper bag.

Put shortening in oblong pan 13 x 9, and set in pre-heated oven at 425 degrees to melt.

Shake 3 or 4 pieces of chicken at a time in bag to coat thoroughly.

Place chicken, skin-side down, in a single layer in the hot shortening.

Bake 30 minutes, then turn skin-side up and bake for 30 minutes more or until chicken is tender.

Makes 4 servings.

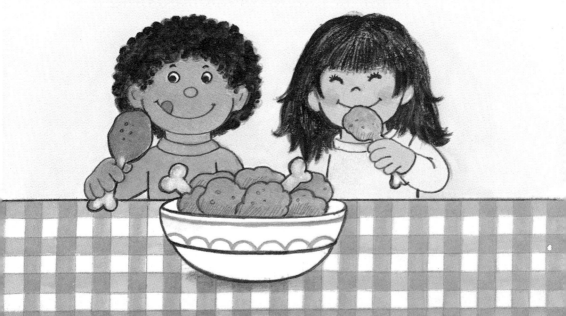

EGGS

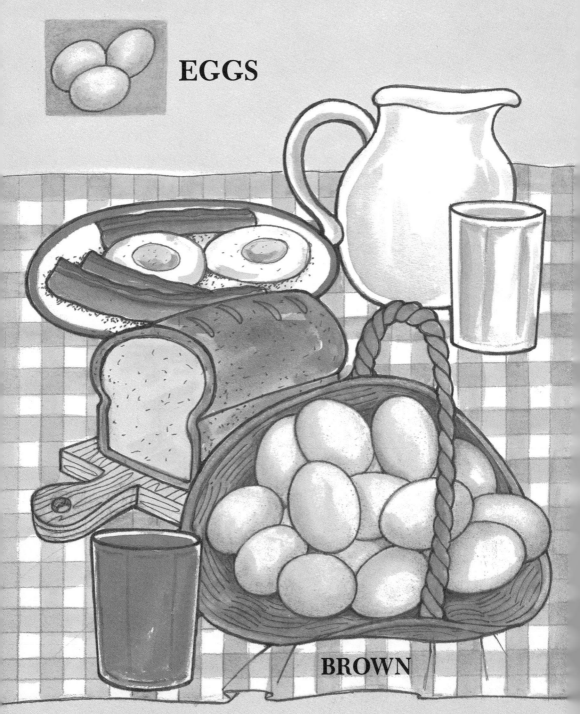

BROWN

Eggs come from chickens.
Egg whites are a good source of protein.
Egg yolks are a good source of iron.

Eggs in a Nest

2 eggs
2 slices of bread
2 tablespoons butter or margarine
Salt and pepper

Cut a circle out of the center of each slice of bread with a round cookie cutter or top of a small glass.

Melt the 2 tablespoons of butter or margarine in a large skillet over medium heat.

Fry bread slices first on one side and then the other.

Turn heat down low, then break one egg into the hole in each piece of bread.

Sprinkle with salt and pepper.

Cover and cook for 3 to 5 minutes.

Makes 2 servings.

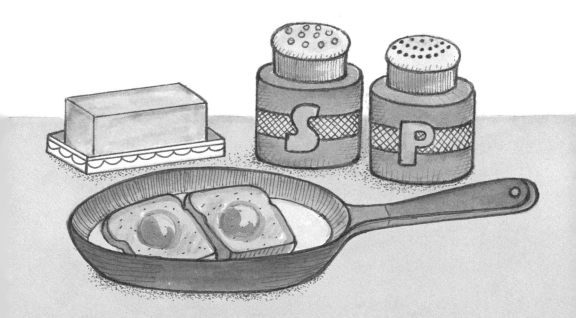

PROTEIN BUILDING BLOCKS

Proteins are made of building blocks called amino acids.

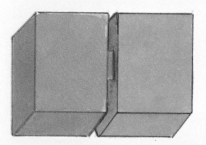

Protein from meat, poultry, and fish has all the building blocks our bodies need.

It is called complete protein.

Complete protein builds and repairs our bodies.

Complete protein is important to help us grow and stay healthy.

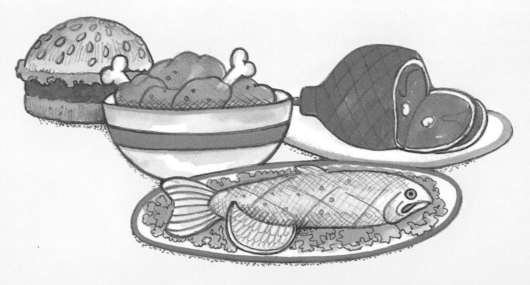

Protein from plants is called "incomplete protein."

It does not have all the building blocks that our bodies need.

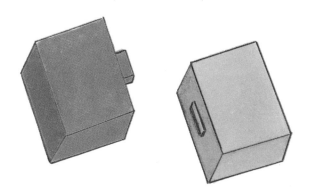

When we eat certain incomplete protein foods together, they join their building blocks to make complete protein in our bodies.

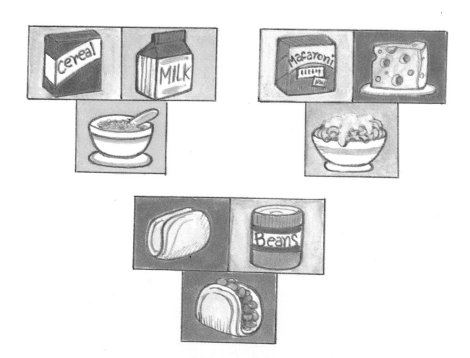

PEANUTS AND
OTHER NUTS

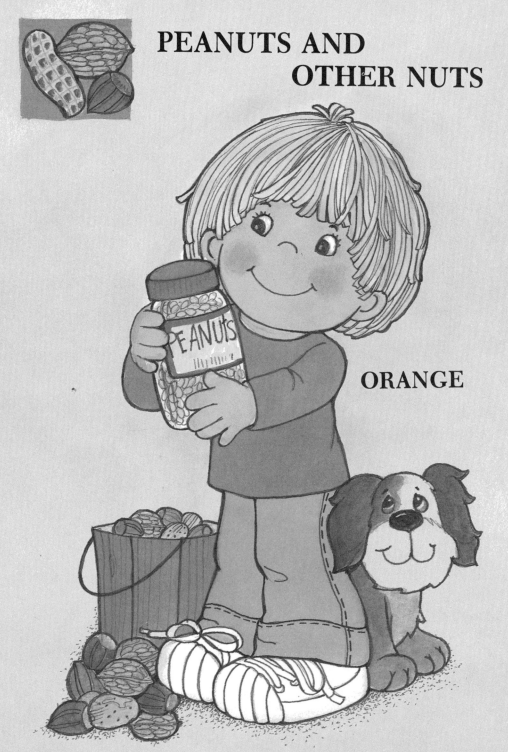

ORANGE

Peanuts are an incomplete source of protein.
Peanut butter on bread makes a complete source of protein.

P B J Party Sandwiches

3 slices of white bread
Peanut butter
Jelly

With a cookie cutter or knife, cut out animal shapes, or shapes you like, from the bread.

Cut three of the same shape for each sandwich.

Spread peanut butter on one bread shape, then put another of the same shaped piece of bread on top.

Spread jelly on top, then cover it with the third piece of shaped bread.

Stand the sandwich on the plate.

Makes 1 serving.

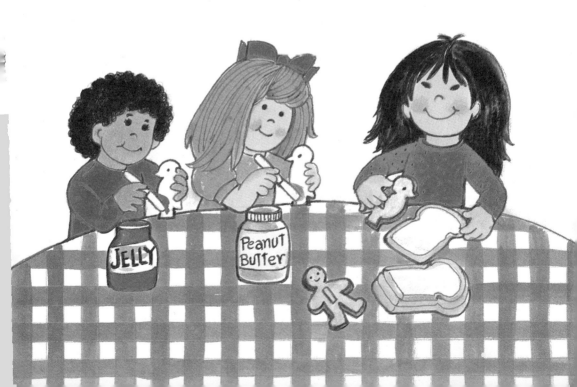

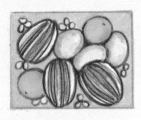

DRY BEANS AND SEEDS
PEAS AND LENTILS

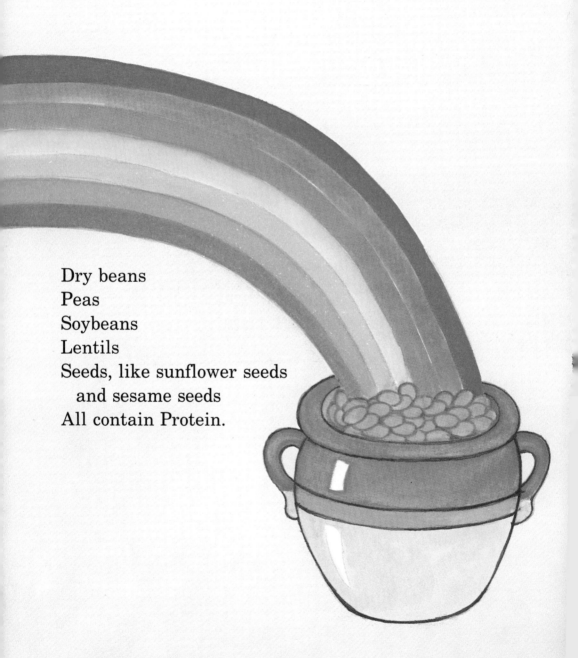

Dry beans
Peas
Soybeans
Lentils
Seeds, like sunflower seeds
  and sesame seeds
All contain Protein.

Baked Beans Casserole

1 18-ounce jar of baked beans
1 tablespoon catsup
1 teaspoon prepared mustard
6 hot dogs

Combine baked beans, catsup, and mustard and pour into oblong baking dish.

Place hot dogs side by side on top.

Bake in a 350 degree oven for 20 minutes, or until hot dogs are browned and bean mixture is bubbly.

Makes 6 servings.

Serving tip: Serve with carrot and celery sticks.

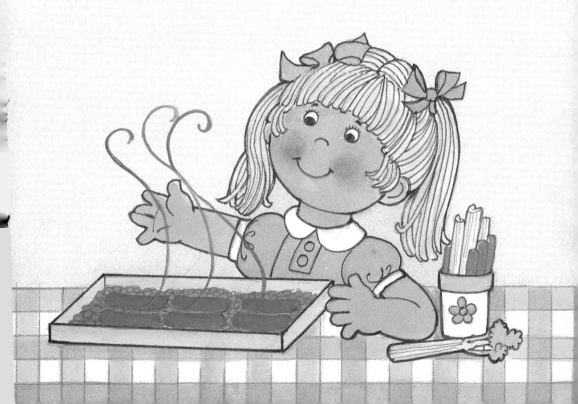

We thank You, God,
for meat to grow on.
Amen.

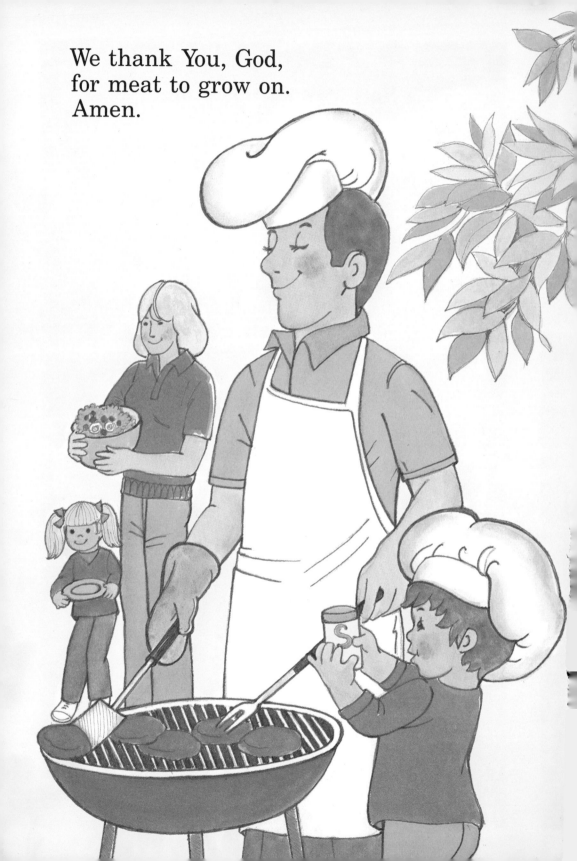